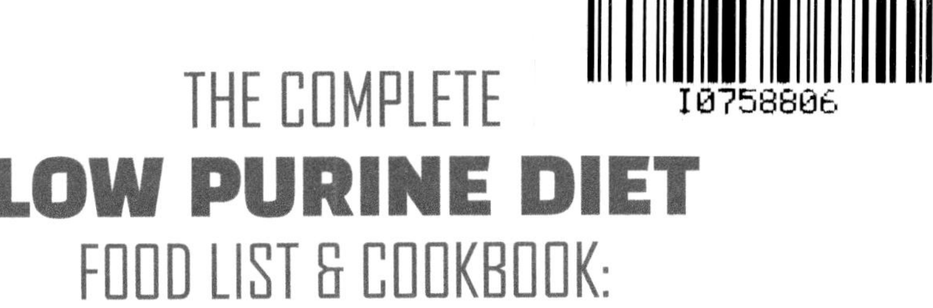

THE COMPLETE
LOW PURINE DIET
FOOD LIST & COOKBOOK:

Delicious Recipes and Tips for Managing Gout.

SARAH ROONEY

First Edition: **March 2023**

TABLE OF CONTENT

INTRODUCTION

I want to start by saying thank you for choosing this book. I hope you found it insightful and helpful.

What is Gout?

Gout is a type of arthritis that occurs when there is a buildup of uric acid crystals in the joints. Uric acid is a waste product that is normally excreted from the body through urine, but in people with gout, the body produces too much uric acid or does not excrete it properly. The excess uric acid forms crystals that accumulate in the joints, causing inflammation, swelling, and pain. Gout typically affects the big toe, but it can also occur in other joints such as the ankle, knee, elbow, wrist, and fingers. Symptoms of gout include sudden and intense pain, redness, warmth, and stiffness in the affected joint. Gout is often managed through lifestyle changes such as a low-purine diet, medication, and other treatments to reduce inflammation and prevent future gout attacks.

How does the Low Purine Diet help manage Gout Symptoms?

A low-purine diet is a dietary approach that can help manage gout symptoms by reducing the number of purines in the diet. Purines are a type of substance found in many foods, and when purines are broken down by the body, uric acid is produced. For people with gout, high levels of uric acid can lead to the formation of uric acid crystals in the joints, causing pain, inflammation, and other symptoms.

By reducing the number of purines in the diet, the low purine diet can help lower the levels of uric acid in the body, reducing the risk of gout attacks and helping to manage existing symptoms. The low purine diet involves avoiding or limiting high-purine foods such as red meat, organ meats (like liver and kidneys), seafood, and some vegetables (like asparagus and mushrooms). Instead, it emphasizes foods that are low in purines, such as whole grains, fruits, vegetables, low-fat dairy products, and lean proteins like chicken and turkey.

In addition to helping manage gout symptoms, the low purine diet may also have other health benefits, such as reducing the risk of heart disease and promoting overall health and wellbeing. However, it's important to note that the low-purine diet is not a cure for gout, and it should be used in conjunction with other treatments and lifestyle changes as recommended by a healthcare professional.

Here is some more information about how the low purine diet helps manage gout symptoms:

When a person with gout consumes high-purine foods, their body produces more uric acid than it can excrete. This leads to a buildup of uric acid in the bloodstream, which can cause urate crystals to form in the joints, leading to inflammation and pain.

The low-purine diet aims to reduce the intake of purines, and therefore reduce the amount of uric acid in the bloodstream. By limiting the consumption of high-purine foods, the body produces less uric acid and there is less uric acid available to form crystals in the joints.

In addition to reducing purine intake, the low-purine diet also encourages the consumption of foods that can help lower uric acid levels in the body. For example, foods that are high in vitamin C (such as citrus fruits, strawberries, and kiwi) can help lower uric acid levels, while foods that are high in complex carbohydrates (such as whole grains, vegetables, and legumes) can help increase the excretion of uric acid from the body.

Overall, the low purine diet is an important part of managing gout symptoms, but it is just one component of a comprehensive treatment plan. Other lifestyle changes, such as maintaining a healthy weight, staying hydrated, and getting regular exercise, can also help reduce the frequency and severity of gout attacks. Additionally, medications such as nonsteroidal anti-inflammatory drugs (NSAIDs), colchicine, and urate-lowering therapies may be prescribed by a healthcare professional to help manage gout symptoms.

My personal story and experience with Gout

I'm a registered dietician with over 10 years of experience helping clients manage their health through nutrition. My passion for nutrition stems from my personal experience with gout, which I was diagnosed with in my mid-30s.

I first began experiencing gout symptoms shortly after the birth of my second child. At first, I thought the pain and swelling in my big toe were due to the physical demands of caring for a newborn. However, as the symptoms persisted, I knew something was wrong. After consulting with my healthcare provider, I was diagnosed with gout and was advised to make lifestyle changes to manage my symptoms.

As a dietician, I was well aware of the connection between diet and gout, and I immediately began researching the low-purine diet. I found that by reducing my intake of high-purine foods and increasing my intake of low-purine foods, I was able to manage my symptoms and reduce the frequency of gout attacks.

Over the years, I have refined my knowledge of the low-purine diet and have helped countless clients with gout manage their symptoms through dietary changes. I understand the challenges of making dietary changes, especially when it comes to giving up favourite foods, and I work with my clients to develop personalized meal plans that are both nutritious and delicious.

My personal experience with gout has given me a unique perspective and a deep understanding of the challenges that people with gout face. I am passionate about helping others manage their symptoms through diet and lifestyle changes and am dedicated to making the journey to better health as smooth and enjoyable as possible.

CHAPTER ONE

UNDERSTANDING PURINES AND GOUT

What exactly are Purines?

Purines are naturally occurring chemicals present in a variety of foods, most notably animal proteins such as meat, fish, and poultry. Purines may also be present in plant-based meals such as beans, lentils, and spinach. As a byproduct of purine breakdown, the body produces uric acid. Uric acid normally dissolves in the blood and is eliminated from the body through the kidneys. In those with gout, however, uric acid accumulates in the blood and may form crystals in the joints, resulting in painful and swollen joints.

What are the effects of Purines on the body?

Purines occur naturally as chemicals present in many foods that play a vital function in the metabolism of the body. As a byproduct of purine breakdown, the body produces uric acid. Uric acid normally dissolves in the blood and is eliminated from the body via the kidneys. In those with gout, however, uric acid accumulates in the blood and may form spikes in the joints, resulting in painful and swollen joints.

Purines may also have additional impacts on the body, such as boosting free radical generation and inflammation. Purine levels in the body that are too high may cause oxidative stress, which can cause cell damage and lead to the growth of chronic illnesses including heart disease and diabetes. Moreover, excessive purine levels may cause the body to manufacture more uric acid than it can eliminate, resulting in uric acid crystal formation and the development of gout.

Besides gout, elevated purine levels in the body may lead to the occurrence of various health problems. High amounts of uric acid in the blood, for example, may increase the chance of developing kidney stones. This is because uric acid may build up in the kidneys and form crystals, leading to the production of kidney stones. Moreover, elevated purine levels have been associated with a greater likelihood of developing heart disease and other inflammatory disorders such as rheumatoid arthritis.

It is important to note, however, that not all purines are harmful. Purines are also crucial building components for DNA and RNA, which are required for biological functions in the body. Purines are required by the body for optimal functioning, therefore a low-purine diet is not suggested for everyone. It is only advised for individuals with a diagnosis of gout or who are at risk of developing it.

As a result, it is critical for persons with gout to maintain a nutritious diet that includes a range of nutrient-dense meals while reducing high-purine foods. This may assist with symptom management and the production of uric acid crystals in the joints. A trained dietician may assist in the development of tailored meal plans and provide advice on how to make healthy food choices while still consuming a variety and tasty diet.

What's the connection between Gout and Purines?

Gout is a kind of arthritis characterized by the buildup of uric acid crystals in the joints, resulting in inflammation and discomfort. Purines are naturally occurring chemicals present in a variety of foods, most notably animal proteins such as meat, fish, and poultry. Purines may also be present in plant-based meals such as beans, lentils, and spinach.

As a byproduct of purine breakdown, the body produces uric acid. Uric acid normally dissolves in the blood and is eliminated from the body through the kidneys. In those with gout, however, uric acid accumulates in the blood and may form crystals in the joints, resulting in painful and swollen joints.

As a result, a diet heavy in purine-rich foods may lead to the development of gout or worsen symptoms in people who already have it. Gout patients are sometimes encouraged to adopt a low-purine diet, which entails restricting or eliminating high-purine foods such as organ meats, seafood, and certain vegetables. This may assist with symptom management and the production of uric acid crystals in the joints. A trained dietician may assist in the development of tailored meal plans and provide advice on how to make nutritious food decisions while still enjoying a variety and tasty diet.

CHAPTER TWO

AN OVERVIEW OF THE LOW PURINE DIET

What exactly is the Low Purine Diet?

The low-purine diet is a type of diet that aims to reduce the consumption of purine-rich foods, which can contribute to the development of gout or aggravate symptoms in those who already have it. Organ meats (liver, kidney, and sweetbreads), red meat, game meat, shellfish, anchovies, sardines, and certain vegetables such as asparagus, spinach, and mushrooms are restricted or avoided in the diet.

Instead, the low-purine diet emphasizes low-purine foods like fruits, vegetables, whole grains, low-fat dairy products, and lean proteins like poultry, fish, and legumes. The low purine diet is not vegetarian or vegan because some plant-based foods, such as lentils and beans, are high in purines.

The goal of the low purine diet is to keep uric acid levels in the blood healthy and to prevent the formation of uric acid crystals in the joints, lowering the risk of gout attacks and managing symptoms in those who already have the condition. A registered dietician can assist in developing a personalized meal plan that meets the nutritional needs of the individual while adhering to the principles of the low-purine diet.

How does the Low Purine Diet help with Gout management?

The low purine diet helps to manage gout by lowering the number of purines in the diet, which reduces the body's production of uric acid. Uric acid is a waste product produced by the body when purines, which are naturally occurring substances found in many foods, are broken down.

Excess uric acid accumulates in the blood of gout patients and can form crystals in the joints, causing inflammation and pain. Individuals can reduce the amount of uric acid produced in the body and help prevent the formation of uric acid crystals in the joints by following a low-purine diet.

High-purine foods such as organ meats, red meat, game meat, shellfish, anchovies, sardines, and certain vegetables are limited or avoided on the low-purine diet. Instead, the diet emphasizes low-purine foods like fruits and vegetables, whole grains, low-fat dairy products, and lean proteins like poultry, fish, and legumes.

In addition to reducing purine intake, the low purine diet also promotes weight loss and a healthy lifestyle, which can help to manage gout symptoms. Losing weight can help to reduce the production of uric acid in the body, while regular exercise can improve joint health and reduce inflammation.

To further clarify how the low purine diet works to control gout, it's vital to understand the function of purines and uric acid in the body. Purines are chemicals present in many meals, and when they are broken down in the body, they form a waste product called uric acid. Uric acid is normally eliminated by the kidneys and expelled in the urine.

Excess uric acid builds in the blood of persons with gout, which may lead to the production of uric acid crystals in the joints. A gout episode is characterized by extreme pain, swelling, and inflammation caused by these crystals.

The low-purine diet works by limiting the consumption of high-purine foods, which helps to reduce uric acid production in the body. Consuming fewer purines causes the body to create less uric acid, which may assist to avoid the production of uric acid crystals in the joints, lowering the frequency and severity of gout episodes.

The low-purine diet is not an exclusion diet, but rather a balanced approach to eating that promotes healthful, low-purine foods. Purine-rich foods, such as organ meats, red meat, seafood, and certain vegetables, are restricted or avoided. Instead, the diet is high in fruits and vegetables, healthy grains, low-fat dairy products, and lean meats like chicken, turkey, fish, and lentils.

Overall, the reduced purine diet is a safe and effective method of managing gout symptoms and lowering the risk of gout episodes. Nevertheless, before making any big changes to your diet or lifestyle, you should contact a healthcare professional or qualified dietitian, particularly if you have other health concerns or are taking medication for gout or other health issues.

The Advantages of a Low Purine Diet

Those with gout or those who want to lower their risk of getting the ailment may benefit from a reduced purine diet. Here are some of the primary advantages of a low-purine diet:

Reduced Gout attacks: One of the most significant advantages of a low purine diet is that it can help to reduce the frequency and severity of gout attacks. Limiting your intake of high-purine foods causes your body to produce less uric acid, which can help to prevent the formation of uric acid crystals in your joints, which causes gout attacks.

Improved Joint Health: A low purine diet can also aid in the improvement of joint health and the reduction of inflammation in the body. The diet can help to reduce joint pain and stiffness associated with gout by reducing the intake of high-purine foods that contribute to inflammation.

Weight Loss: Many high-purine foods are also high in calories and can contribute to weight gain. People can better manage their weight and reduce their risk of developing gout by following a low-purine diet that emphasizes healthy, low-calorie foods.

Increased Heart Health: The low purine diet is also good for your heart since it encourages you to eat heart-healthy foods like fruits, vegetables, whole grains, and lean meats. These meals are high in nutrients that may help decrease blood pressure, cholesterol, and the risk of heart disease.

Increased Nutrient intake: The low purine diet promotes the eating of a broad range of fruits, vegetables, whole grains, and lean meats, which may aid in nutrient intake and general health.

Better digestion: Several high-purine meals may be difficult to digest, contributing to digestive issues including bloating and constipation. The low-purine diet may assist to enhance digestive health by limiting your consumption of these items and concentrating on low-purine, high-fibre meals.

Overall, the reduced purine diet has a lot of advantages for persons who have gout or want to lower their chance of getting it. Individuals may control their gout symptoms, improve their general health, and lower their risk of associated illnesses such as heart disease and obesity by adopting a balanced, low-purine eating plan.

How to Begin and Maintain a Low Purine Diet

Beginning and sticking to a low-purine diet might be difficult, but there are a few tricks that can make the process simpler and more successful:

Consult a Medical Professional: It is important to talk with a healthcare practitioner before beginning any new diet or making any changes to your eating habits. A dietician or nutritionist may assist you in developing a meal plan that matches your specific requirements and ensures you are receiving all of the required nutrients.

Inform yourself about Purine-Rich Foods: To be effective on the low-purine diet, you must first understand which foods are rich in purines and should be restricted or avoided. Organ meats, shellfish, and some vegetables such as mushrooms and asparagus are examples of high-purine foods.

Plan your Meals: Preparing your meals ahead of time might help you keep to the reduced purine diet and prevent temptation. Make a weekly food plan, and a shopping list, and plan ahead of time to cook meals and snacks.

Concentrate on Low-Purine, High-fiber Foods: During meal planning, prioritize foods low in purines and rich in fibre. Fruits, vegetables, whole grains, and lean meats like chicken or turkey are all good choices.

Drink lots of Water: Water may help remove excess uric acid from the body and avoid gout episodes. Aim for 8 to 10 glasses of water every day.

Limit or avoid Alcohol: Since it raises uric acid levels in the body, alcohol may contribute to gout episodes. Reducing or eliminating alcohol consumption may help control gout symptoms.

Keep track of your progress: Keep note of your gout symptoms and how you're doing with the reduced purine diet. If you aren't seeing results, you may need to change your diet or seek further guidance from a healthcare practitioner.

Ultimately, the key to beginning and sticking to a low-purine diet is to educate yourself, plan your meals ahead of time, and concentrate on a healthy, balanced diet rich in fibre and low in purines. You may effectively manage your gout symptoms and improve your overall health by following these suggestions and consulting with a healthcare expert.

CHAPTER THREE

LOW PURINE FOODS LIST

Introduction to Low Purine Foods

The low purine diet is a sort of eating plan that seeks to lower purine levels in the body, which may assist with illnesses including gout and kidney stones. Purines are naturally occurring chemicals present in a variety of foods that, when broken down in the body, generate uric acid. Uric acid levels that are too high might cause crystals to develop in the joints, causing discomfort, inflammation, and oedema.

The low-purine diet comprises restricting or eliminating purine-rich foods such as organ meats, shellfish, and certain vegetables. Instead, the diet emphasizes low-purine foods such as fruits, vegetables, healthy grains, and lean meats.

A low purine diet reduces the likelihood of gout episodes, reduces inflammation, and improves kidney function. It is crucial to highlight, however, that the reduced purine diet is not a one-size-fits-all solution and should be adapted to individual requirements and medical circumstances.

You may assist control your gout symptoms and enhance your general health by introducing more low-purine foods into your diet and avoiding high-purine meals. Working with a healthcare expert or a dietitian to establish a tailored meal plan that suits your specific requirements and objectives is essential.

Food List

here is a comprehensive list of low-purine foods organized by food group:

Fruits and Vegetables

Apples

Bananas

Berries (strawberries, blueberries, raspberries, etc.)

Cherries

Citrus fruits (oranges, lemons, limes, etc.)

Grapes

Melons (watermelon, cantaloupe, honeydew, etc.)

Pears

Pineapple

Avocado

Bell peppers

Broccoli

Cabbage

Carrots

Cauliflower

Cucumbers

Eggplant

Green beans

Lettuce and leafy greens (spinach, kale, arugula, etc.)

Mushrooms

Onions

Peas

Potatoes

Tomatoes

Zucchini

Grains and Starches

Bread (white or whole grain)

Cereal (oatmeal, corn flakes, etc.)

Pasta (white or whole grain)

Rice (white or brown)

Quinoa

Barley

Bulgur

Meat and Meat Alternatives

Chicken (skinless)

Turkey (skinless)

Lean cuts of beef (round, sirloin, tenderloin)

Pork (tenderloin)

Tofu

Beans (black, kidney, navy, etc.)

Lentils

Dairy and Dairy Alternatives

Milk (skim or low-fat)

Cheese (low-fat)

Yoghurt (low-fat)

Fats and Oils

Olive oil

Canola oil

Avocado oil

Although these foods are typically low in purines, the actual purine concentration might vary based on variables such as processing, cooking techniques, and individual tolerance. Working with a healthcare expert or a dietitian to establish a tailored meal plan that suits your specific requirements and objectives is always a smart idea.

CHAPTER FOUR

DELICIOUS LOW-PURINE RECIPES

Breakfast Recipes

Here are ten healthy and delicious recipes that are low in purines and suitable for someone following a low-purine diet:

Quinoa Salad with Roasted Vegetables and Lemon Vinaigrette

Ingredients:

1 cup quinoa

2 cups water

2 medium zucchini, sliced into rounds

1 red bell pepper, seeded and chopped

1 yellow bell pepper, seeded and chopped

1 red onion, chopped

2 tablespoons olive oil

1/2 teaspoon salt

1/4 teaspoon black pepper

1/4 cup fresh parsley, chopped

1/4 cup fresh mint, chopped

2 tablespoons lemon juice

1 tablespoon honey

Instructions:

Preheat the oven to 425°F (220°C).

Rinse the quinoa and place it in a medium saucepan with water. Bring to a boil, then reduce the heat to low and simmer for 15-20 minutes, or until the water is absorbed and the quinoa is tender.

While the quinoa is cooking, place the zucchini, bell peppers, and red onion on a large baking sheet. Drizzle with olive oil and sprinkle with salt and black pepper. Toss to coat.

Roast the vegetables in the oven for 20-25 minutes, or until tender and lightly browned.

In a small bowl, whisk together the lemon juice and honey to make the vinaigrette.

In a large bowl, combine the cooked quinoa, roasted vegetables, parsley, and mint. Drizzle with the lemon vinaigrette and toss to coat.

Serve the quinoa salad warm or at room temperature.

Nutritional information per serving:

Calories: 267

Fat: 9g

Carbohydrates: 41g

Fibre: 6g

Protein: 8g

Baked Salmon with Herb Butter and Asparagus

Ingredients:

4 salmon fillets (4-6 ounces each)

1 pound asparagus, trimmed

2 tablespoons olive oil

Salt and pepper, to taste

4 tablespoons unsalted butter, softened

1 tablespoon chopped fresh dill

1 tablespoon chopped fresh parsley

1 garlic clove, minced

Instructions:

Preheat the oven to 400°F (200°C).

Line a baking sheet with parchment paper.

Arrange the salmon fillets and asparagus on the baking sheet. Drizzle with olive oil and sprinkle with salt and pepper.

In a small bowl, combine the softened butter, dill, parsley, and garlic. Mix well.

Place a dollop of the herb butter on each salmon fillet.

Bake the salmon and asparagus in the oven for 12-15 minutes, or until the salmon is cooked through and the asparagus is tender.

Serve the baked salmon and asparagus hot.

Nutritional information per serving:

Calories: 354

Fat: 26g

Carbohydrates: 5g

Fibre: 2g

Protein: 26g

Grilled Lemon Garlic Chicken with Zucchini

Ingredients:

4 boneless, skinless chicken breasts

2 lemons, juiced

2 cloves garlic, minced

2 tablespoons olive oil

1 teaspoon dried oregano

Salt and pepper, to taste

4 medium zucchinis, sliced

Instructions:

Preheat the grill to medium-high heat.

In a small bowl, whisk together the lemon juice, minced garlic, olive oil, dried oregano, salt, and pepper.

Place the chicken breasts in a large resealable plastic bag and pour in the marinade. Seal the bag and toss it to coat the chicken evenly. Let marinate in the refrigerator for at least 30 minutes.

While the chicken is marinating, prepare the zucchini. Slice each zucchini into ¼-inch thick rounds.

Once the grill is heated, remove the chicken from the marinade and discard the remaining marinade. Grill the chicken for 5-6 minutes per side or until cooked through.

While the chicken is grilling, add the sliced zucchini to a grill pan or grill basket. Grill for 3-4 minutes per side or until tender and lightly charred.

Serve the grilled chicken with the grilled zucchini on the side.

Nutritional Information:

Calories: 312

Fat: 12g

Protein: 43g

Carbohydrates: 6g

Fibre: 2g

Sodium: 153mg

Note: This recipe is low in purines and high in protein, making it a great option for those on a low-purine diet. The grilled zucchini is a delicious and healthy side dish that complements the lemon garlic flavour of the chicken.

Banana Oat Pancakes

Ingredients:

1 cup rolled oats

2 ripe bananas, mashed

2 eggs

1 teaspoon vanilla extract

½ teaspoon ground cinnamon

1 teaspoon baking powder

¼ teaspoon salt

1 tablespoon honey

Cooking spray

Instructions:

In a blender, combine the rolled oats, mashed bananas, eggs, vanilla extract, cinnamon, baking powder, salt, and honey. Blend until smooth.

Heat a non-stick skillet or griddle over medium heat. Spray with cooking spray.

Pour ¼ cup of batter onto the skillet for each pancake.

Cook until bubbles form on the surface of the pancake, then flip and cook until golden brown.

Serve warm with fresh fruit and a drizzle of honey.

Nutritional Information:

Calories: 342

Fat: 7g

Protein: 13g

Carbohydrates: 62g

Fibre: 8g

Sodium: 385mg

Egg White and Veggie Breakfast Scramble

Ingredients:

6 egg whites

1 cup chopped mixed vegetables (such as bell pepper, onion, and spinach)

1 tablespoon olive oil

Salt and pepper, to taste

2 slices whole-grain toast

Instructions:

Heat the olive oil in a non-stick skillet over medium heat.

Add the chopped mixed vegetables and cook until softened.

Pour in the egg whites and cook, stirring occasionally, until fully cooked.

Season with salt and pepper to taste.

Serve hot with 2 slices of whole grain toast.

Nutritional Information:

Calories: 225

Fat: 7g

Protein: 17g

Carbohydrates: 23g

Fibre: 5g

Sodium: 394mg

Greek Yogurt Parfait

Ingredients:

1 cup plain Greek yoghurt

½ cup fresh berries (such as blueberries or strawberries)

¼ cup chopped nuts (such as almonds or walnuts)

1 tablespoon honey

Instructions:

Layer the Greek yoghurt, fresh berries, and chopped nuts in a bowl or parfait glass.

Drizzle with honey.

Serve chilled.

Nutritional Information:

Calories: 310

Fat: 17g

Protein: 22g

Carbohydrates: 20g

Fibre: 3g

Sodium: 47mg

Spinach and Feta Breakfast Wrap

Ingredients:

1 large whole-grain wrap

2 eggs

½ cup fresh spinach leaves

2 tablespoons crumbled feta cheese

Salt and pepper, to taste

Instructions:

Whisk the eggs in a small bowl and season with salt
and pepper.

Heat a non-stick skillet over medium heat.

Add the whisked eggs and spinach leaves to the skillet and cook until the eggs are fully cooked and the spinach is wilted.

Spoon the cooked eggs and spinach onto the centre of the whole-grain wrap.

Sprinkle the crumbled feta cheese over the eggs and spinach.

Fold the edges of the wrap inwards to create a burrito-style wrap.

Serve hot.

Nutritional Information:

Calories: 345

Fat: 16g

Protein: 22g

Carbohydrates: 29g

Fibre: 8g

Sodium: 652mg

Spinach and Mushroom Omelette

Ingredients:

2 eggs

1 cup spinach leaves, chopped

1/2 cup mushrooms, sliced

1/4 cup onion, chopped

1/4 cup shredded cheddar cheese

Salt and pepper to taste

1 tsp olive oil

Instructions:

In a nonstick skillet, heat the olive oil over medium heat.

Add the onion and mushrooms, and cook for 3-5 minutes, until they are tender.

Add the spinach to the skillet and cook until wilted.

In a small bowl, whisk the eggs with salt and pepper.

Pour the eggs over the vegetables in the skillet and sprinkle the shredded cheese on top.

Cook the omelette for 2-3 minutes, until the bottom, is set and the top is slightly runny.

Use a spatula to fold the omelette in half and cook for another 1-2 minutes, until the cheese is melted and the eggs are fully cooked.

Serve hot with toast or fruit on the side.

Nutritional Information:

Calories: 320

Protein: 22g

Carbohydrates: 7g

Fat: 24g

Fibre: 2g

Sodium: 390mg

Greek Yogurt Parfait

Ingredients:

1 cup plain Greek yoghurt

1/4 cup fresh berries (blueberries, raspberries, or strawberries)

1/4 cup granola

1 tbsp honey

Instructions:

In a small glass or bowl, layer the yoghurt, berries, and granola.

Drizzle the honey over the top.

Serve cold as a breakfast or snack.

Nutritional Information:

Calories: 290

Protein: 20g

Carbohydrates: 37g

Fat: 7g

Fibre: 4g

Sodium: 70mg

Sweet Potato and Egg Breakfast Skillet

Ingredients:

1 large sweet potato, peeled and diced

1/2 cup bell pepper, chopped

1/2 cup onion, chopped

2 cloves garlic, minced

2 eggs

1 tbsp olive oil

Salt and pepper to taste

Instructions:

In a large skillet, heat the olive oil over medium heat.

Add the sweet potato, bell pepper, onion, and garlic to the skillet, and cook for 8-10 minutes, until the vegetables are tender.

Crack the eggs over the vegetables and season with salt and pepper.

Cover the skillet and cook for another 3-5 minutes, until the eggs are cooked to your desired doneness.

Serve hot as a breakfast or brunch.

Nutritional Information:

Calories: 350

Protein: 12g

Carbohydrates: 38g

Fat: 18g

Fibre: 6g

Sodium: 190mg

Greek Salad with Grilled Chicken

Ingredients:

1 lb boneless, skinless chicken breasts

2 tbsp olive oil

1 tsp dried oregano

Salt and pepper to taste

1 head romaine lettuce, chopped

1 cup cherry tomatoes, halved

1 small red onion, sliced

1 small cucumber, chopped

½ cup crumbled feta cheese

¼ cup pitted kalamata olives

For the dressing:

¼ cup olive oil

2 tbsp red wine vinegar

1 tsp dried oregano

Salt and pepper to taste

Instructions:

Preheat a grill or grill pan to medium-high heat.

In a small bowl, mix the olive oil, oregano, salt, and pepper. Brush the chicken breasts with the mixture and place them on the grill. Cook for 6-7 minutes per side or until the internal temperature reaches 165°F.

In a large bowl, combine the romaine lettuce, cherry tomatoes, red onion, and cucumber.

In a small bowl, whisk together the olive oil, red wine vinegar, oregano, salt, and pepper to make the dressing.

Once the chicken is cooked, let it rest for 5 minutes before slicing it into strips.

Add the chicken strips, feta cheese, and olives to the bowl with the salad ingredients. Toss with the dressing and serve immediately.

Nutrition Facts:

Servings: 4 | Serving size: 1/4 recipe

Calories: 400 | Total Fat: 28g | Saturated Fat: 6g |

Carbohydrates: 9g | Fiber: 3g | Sugar: 5g | Protein:

29g | Sodium: 720mg

Quinoa Veggie Bowl

Ingredients:

1 cup quinoa

2 cups vegetable broth

1 small sweet potato, cubed

1 small zucchini, chopped

1 red bell pepper, chopped

1 yellow bell pepper, chopped

1 cup cherry tomatoes, halved

1 can chickpeas, drained and rinsed

2 tbsp olive oil

1 tsp ground cumin

Salt and pepper to taste

For the dressing:

¼ cup olive oil

2 tbsp lemon juice

1 garlic clove, minced

Salt and pepper to taste

Instructions:

Rinse the quinoa under cold water and drain. In a medium saucepan, combine the quinoa and vegetable broth. Bring to a boil, then reduce heat to low and simmer for 15-20 minutes, or until the quinoa is tender.

Preheat the oven to 400°F.

Spread the sweet potato, zucchini, and bell peppers on a baking sheet. Drizzle with olive oil and sprinkle with cumin, salt, and pepper. Roast for 20-25 minutes, or until the vegetables are tender.

In a small bowl, whisk together the olive oil, lemon juice, garlic, salt, and pepper to make the dressing.

Once the quinoa and vegetables are cooked, divide the quinoa among four bowls. Top with roasted vegetables, cherry tomatoes, and chickpeas. Drizzle with the dressing and serve immediately.

Nutrition Facts:

Servings: 4 | Serving size: 1/4 recipe

Calories: 380 | Total Fat: 19g | Saturated Fat: 3g |

 Carbohydrates: 44g | Fiber:

Greek Quinoa Salad

Ingredients:

1 cup quinoa

2 cups water

1/2 cup chopped red onion

1/2 cup chopped cucumber

1/2 cup chopped bell pepper

1/2 cup cherry tomatoes, halved

1/4 cup crumbled feta cheese

1/4 cup chopped fresh parsley

1/4 cup chopped fresh mint

3 tablespoons olive oil

2 tablespoons lemon juice

Salt and pepper to taste

Instructions:

Rinse the quinoa thoroughly and place it in a pot with

 2 cups of water. Bring to a boil, then reduce heat

and simmer for 15-20 minutes or until the water is absorbed and the quinoa is tender.

In a large bowl, combine the cooked quinoa with the red onion, cucumber, bell pepper, cherry tomatoes, feta cheese, parsley, and mint.

In a small bowl, whisk together the olive oil, lemon juice, salt, and pepper. Pour the dressing over the quinoa salad and toss to coat. Serve chilled.

Nutrition facts per serving (serves 4):

Calories: 290

Fat: 16g

Carbohydrates: 29g

Protein: 8g

Fibre: 5g

Chickpea and Avocado Salad

Ingredients:

1 can chickpeas, drained and rinsed

1 avocado, diced

1/2 cup chopped red onion

1/2 cup chopped cucumber

1/2 cup cherry tomatoes, halved

2 tablespoons chopped fresh cilantro

2 tablespoons olive oil

1 tablespoon lemon juice

Salt and pepper to taste

Instructions:

In a large bowl, combine the chickpeas, avocado, red onion, cucumber, cherry tomatoes, and cilantro. In a small bowl, whisk together the olive oil, lemon juice, salt, and pepper. Pour the dressing over the salad and toss to coat. Serve chilled.

Nutrition facts per serving (serves 2):

Calories: 370

Fat: 26g

Carbohydrates: 29g

Protein: 8g

Fibre: 12g

Turkey and Hummus Wrap

Ingredients:

1 large whole wheat wrap

3 ounces sliced turkey

2 tablespoons hummus

1/4 cup chopped cucumber

1/4 cup chopped red onion

1/4 cup shredded lettuce

Instructions:

Lay the wrap flat on a plate or cutting board.

Spread the hummus evenly over the centre of the wrap.

Arrange the turkey, cucumber, red onion, and lettuce on top of the hummus.

Roll the wrap tightly, tucking in the sides as you go. Slice in half and serve.

Nutrition facts per serving (serves 1):

Calories: 330

Fat: 10g

Carbohydrates: 35g

Protein: 26g

Fibre: 6g

Baked Sweet Potato with Black Bean Salsa

Ingredients:

2 medium sweet potatoes

1 can black beans, rinsed and drained

1 small red onion, diced

1 red bell pepper, diced

1 jalapeño pepper, seeded and minced

1 lime, juiced

1/4 cup chopped fresh cilantro

Salt and pepper to taste

Instructions:

Preheat the oven to 400°F.

Scrub the sweet potatoes clean and poke a few holes in them with a fork. Place them on a baking sheet and bake for 45-50 minutes, or until tender.

While the sweet potatoes are baking, prepare the black bean salsa. In a medium bowl, combine the rinsed and drained black beans, diced red onion, diced red bell pepper, minced jalapeño pepper, lime juice, chopped fresh cilantro, salt, and pepper.

When the sweet potatoes are done, remove them from the oven and slice them open lengthwise. Top each sweet potato with a generous scoop of black bean salsa.

Serve hot.

Nutrition Facts:

Calories: 322

Fat: 0.8g

Carbohydrates: 69.1g

Fibre: 17.6g

Protein: 14.5g

Grilled Chicken and Veggie Kabobs

Ingredients:

2 boneless, skinless chicken breasts, cut into bite-sized
 pieces

1 red onion, cut into bite-sized pieces

1 red bell pepper, cut into bite-sized pieces

1 zucchini, sliced into rounds

8-10 cherry tomatoes

1/4 cup olive oil

2 tablespoons balsamic vinegar

2 cloves garlic, minced

Salt and pepper to taste

Instructions:

Preheat the grill to medium-high heat.

Thread the chicken, red onion, red bell pepper, zucchini, and cherry tomatoes onto skewers.

In a small bowl, whisk together the olive oil, balsamic vinegar, minced garlic, salt, and pepper to make the marinade.

Brush the marinade over the chicken and veggies, making sure to coat them well.

Grill the kabobs for 10-12 minutes, or until the chicken is cooked through and the veggies are tender.

Serve hot.

Nutrition Facts:

Calories: 302

Fat: 16.2g

Carbohydrates: 10.7g

Quinoa Salad with Roasted Vegetables

Ingredients:

1 cup quinoa

2 cups water

2 cups mixed vegetables (carrots, broccoli, zucchini)

1 tbsp olive oil

Salt and pepper

1/4 cup chopped fresh parsley

1/4 cup chopped fresh mint

1/4 cup chopped fresh basil

1/4 cup chopped almonds

1/4 cup feta cheese

2 tbsp lemon juice

1 tbsp honey

Instructions:

Preheat the oven to 400°F.

Rinse the quinoa under cold water and place it in a pot with 2 cups of water. Bring to a boil, then reduce the heat to low and cover. Cook for 15-20 minutes, until the water, is absorbed and the quinoa is tender.

Cut the vegetables into small pieces and place them on a baking sheet. Drizzle with olive oil, salt, and pepper. Roast for 20-25 minutes, until tender and slightly charred.

In a large bowl, mix the cooked quinoa, roasted vegetables, chopped herbs, almonds, and feta cheese.

In a small bowl, whisk together the lemon juice and honey. Drizzle over the salad and toss to combine.

Serve the salad immediately, or store it in an airtight container in the refrigerator for up to 3 days.

Nutrition facts per serving (serves 4):

Calories: 320

Total fat: 15g

Saturated fat: 3g

Cholesterol: 8mg

Sodium: 185mg

Total carbohydrates: 40g

Dietary fibre: 7g

Sugar: 9g

Protein: 11g

Greek Yogurt Chicken Salad

Ingredients:

2 cups cooked shredded chicken

1/2 cup plain Greek yoghurt

1/4 cup diced celery

1/4 cup diced red onion

1/4 cup chopped fresh parsley

1/4 cup chopped fresh dill

1/4 cup chopped fresh chives

1 tbsp lemon juice

Salt and pepper

Whole grain bread or lettuce leaves, for serving

Instructions:

In a large bowl, mix the shredded chicken, Greek yoghurt, celery, red onion, parsley, dill, chives, and lemon juice. Season with salt and pepper to taste.

Serve the chicken salad on whole grain bread or lettuce leaves.

Nutrition facts per serving (serves 4):

Calories: 190

Total fat: 5g

Saturated fat: 1g

Cholesterol: 68mg

Sodium: 190mg

Total carbohydrates: 4g

Dietary fibre: 1g

Sugar: 2g

Protein: 31g

Quinoa and Black Bean Salad

Ingredients:

1 cup cooked quinoa

1 can black beans, drained and rinsed

1/2 cup chopped red onion

1/2 cup chopped red bell pepper

1/2 cup chopped cucumber

1/4 cup chopped fresh cilantro

2 tablespoons lime juice

1 tablespoon olive oil

Salt and pepper to taste

Instructions:

In a large mixing bowl, combine cooked quinoa, black beans, red onion, red bell pepper, cucumber, and cilantro.

In a small mixing bowl, whisk together lime juice, olive oil, salt, and pepper.

Pour dressing over the quinoa mixture and toss to combine.

Serve chilled.

Nutrition Facts (per serving):

Calories: 248

Fat: 6g

Carbohydrates: 39g

Protein: 10g

Fibre: 10g

Sugar: 2g

Sodium: 211mg

Baked Salmon with Roasted Vegetables

Ingredients:

4 salmon fillets

1 lb. Brussels sprouts, trimmed and halved

1 red bell pepper, seeded and chopped

1 yellow onion, chopped

2 tablespoons olive oil

Salt and pepper to taste

1 lemon, sliced

Instructions:

Preheat the oven to 400°F.

In a large mixing bowl, combine Brussels sprouts, red bell pepper, and onion. Toss with olive oil, salt, and pepper.

Arrange the vegetables on a large baking sheet.

Season salmon fillets with salt and pepper, and place them on top of the vegetables.

Place lemon slices on top of each salmon fillet.

Bake for 15-20 minutes or until the salmon is cooked through.

Nutrition Facts (per serving):

Calories: 360

Fat: 20g

Carbohydrates: 12g

Protein: 34g

Fibre: 5g

Sugar: 3g

Sodium: 163mg

Mushroom and Spinach Risotto

Ingredients:

1 cup Arborio rice

4 cups low-sodium chicken broth

1 tablespoon olive oil

1/2 cup chopped onion

1 garlic clove, minced

8 oz. mushrooms, sliced

2 cups baby spinach

1/4 cup grated Parmesan cheese

Salt and pepper to taste

Instructions:

In a medium saucepan, bring the chicken broth to a simmer.

In a large saucepan, heat olive oil over medium heat.

Add onion and garlic and sauté for 2-3 minutes.

Add mushrooms and sauté until tender, about 5-7 minutes.

Add Arborio rice and stir for 1-2 minutes until lightly toasted.

Begin adding chicken broth, 1 cup at a time, stirring constantly until the liquid is absorbed before adding the next cup.

Once all the broth has been added and absorbed, stir in baby spinach and Parmesan cheese.

Season with salt and pepper to taste.

Nutrition Facts (per serving):

Calories: 299

Fat: 6g

Carbohydrates: 47g

Protein: 12g

Fibre: 3g

Sugar: 2g / Sodium: 241mg

Turkey and Vegetable Stir-Fry

Ingredients:

1 lb. turkey breast, cut into thin strips

1 red bell pepper, seeded and sliced

1 yellow onion, sliced

2 cups broccoli florets

2 garlic cloves, minced

2 tablespoons low-sodium soy sauce

1 tablespoon cornstarch

1/4 cup water

2 tablespoons vegetable oil

Instructions:

In a small mixing bowl, whisk together soy sauce, cornstarch, and water.

Heat vegetable oil in a large wok or frying pan over high heat.

Add turkey strips and stir-fry for 3-4 minutes until browned.

Add red bell pepper, yellow onion, broccoli, and garlic to the pan.

Stir-fry for 5-7 minutes until vegetables are tender-crisp.

Add the soy sauce mixture to the pan and stir-fry for an additional 2-3 minutes until the sauce has thickened.

Nutrition Facts (per serving):

Calories: 298

Grilled Chicken with Mixed Vegetables

Ingredients:

4 boneless, skinless chicken breasts

1 cup cherry tomatoes

1 cup bell pepper, sliced

1 cup zucchini, sliced

2 tablespoons olive oil

Salt and pepper to taste

Instructions:

Preheat the grill to medium-high heat.

In a bowl, mix the cherry tomatoes, bell pepper, and zucchini with olive oil, salt, and pepper.

Season the chicken breasts with salt and pepper.

Grill the chicken for 6-8 minutes on each side, or until fully cooked.

Grill the mixed vegetables for 4-5 minutes, or until tender.

Nutrition facts (per serving):

Calories: 250

Fat: 10g

Protein: 32g

Carbohydrates: 7g

Fibre: 2g

Quinoa Stuffed Bell Peppers

Ingredients:

4 bell peppers, tops removed and seeded

1 cup quinoa, cooked

1 cup black beans, rinsed and drained

1 cup diced tomatoes

1 cup corn

1/2 cup chopped onion

2 cloves garlic, minced

1 tablespoon olive oil

1 teaspoon cumin

Salt and pepper to taste

Instructions:

Preheat the oven to 375°F (190°C).

In a pan, sauté the onion and garlic in olive oil until translucent.

Add the cooked quinoa, black beans, diced tomatoes, corn, cumin, salt, and pepper to the pan and stir to combine.

Stuff the mixture into the bell peppers.

Place the stuffed peppers in a baking dish and bake in the preheated oven for 30-35 minutes, or until the peppers are tender.

Nutrition facts (per serving):

Calories: 310

Fat: 7g

Protein: 12g

Carbohydrates: 54g

Fibre: 12g

Grilled Lemon Herb Chicken with Roasted Vegetables

Ingredients:

4 boneless, skinless chicken breasts

1/4 cup lemon juice

2 tablespoons olive oil

1 tablespoon chopped fresh thyme

1 tablespoon chopped fresh rosemary

1 teaspoon minced garlic

Salt and black pepper to taste

1 large sweet potato, cubed

1 large red bell pepper, sliced

1 large yellow squash, sliced

1 large zucchini, sliced

Instructions:

In a bowl, whisk together the lemon juice, olive oil, thyme, rosemary, garlic, salt, and black pepper.

Place the chicken breasts in a resealable plastic bag and pour in the marinade. Seal the bag and refrigerate for at least 30 minutes.

Preheat the grill to medium-high heat.

Remove the chicken from the marinade and discard the remaining marinade.

Grill the chicken for 5-6 minutes per side or until cooked through.

Meanwhile, preheat the oven to 400°F.

In a large bowl, toss together the sweet potato, red bell pepper, yellow squash, zucchini, and a drizzle of olive oil. Season with salt and black pepper to taste.

Spread the vegetables out in a single layer on a baking sheet and roast for 20-25 minutes or until tender and slightly caramelized.

Serve the grilled chicken with the roasted vegetables.

Nutrition facts per serving:

Calories: 347

Fat: 11g

Carbohydrates: 28g

Fibre: 6g

Protein: 36g

Baked Salmon with Quinoa and Steamed Asparagus

Ingredients:

4 salmon fillets (4-6 oz each)

1/4 cup Dijon mustard

1 tablespoon honey

1 teaspoon minced garlic

1 teaspoon dried dill

Salt and black pepper to taste

1 cup quinoa, rinsed

2 cups low-sodium vegetable broth

1 pound asparagus, trimmed

1 tablespoon olive oil

Instructions:

Preheat the oven to 375°F.

In a bowl, whisk together the Dijon mustard, honey, garlic, dill, salt, and black pepper.

Place the salmon fillets in a baking dish and brush the mustard mixture over the top of each fillet.

Bake the salmon for 12-15 minutes or until cooked through.

Meanwhile, in a saucepan, bring the quinoa and vegetable broth to a boil. Reduce the heat to low and simmer for 15-20 minutes or until the quinoa is tender and the liquid is absorbed.

In a steamer basket, steam the asparagus for 3-4 minutes or until tender.

Drizzle the asparagus with olive oil and season with salt and black pepper to taste.

Serve the baked salmon with quinoa and steamed asparagus.

Nutrition facts per serving:

Calories: 423

Fat: 16g

Carbohydrates: 35g

Fibre: 6g

Protein: 35g

Lentil Shepherd's Pie.

Ingredients:

2 cups cooked lentils

1 onion, chopped

2 cloves garlic, minced

2 carrots, peeled and diced

2 stalks of celery, diced

1 cup frozen peas

1 cup vegetable broth

2 tablespoons tomato paste

2 teaspoons Worcestershire sauce

1 teaspoon dried thyme

1 teaspoon dried rosemary

Salt and pepper to taste

4 cups mashed potatoes

Instructions:

Preheat oven to 350°F.

In a large skillet, heat a tablespoon of oil over medium heat. Add the onion and garlic and sauté until the onion is translucent.

Add the carrots and celery and continue to cook until they begin to soften.

Add the cooked lentils, peas, vegetable broth, tomato paste, Worcestershire sauce, thyme, rosemary, salt, and pepper to the skillet. Stir to combine.

Reduce heat to low and simmer for 10-15 minutes until the sauce has thickened.

Transfer the lentil mixture to a large baking dish and spread it out in an even layer.

Top the lentil mixture with the mashed potatoes, spreading them out evenly to cover the lentil mixture.

Bake in the preheated oven for 25-30 minutes or until the potatoes are golden brown and the filling is heated through.

Let the shepherd's pie cool for a few minutes before serving.

Nutrition Facts (per serving):

Calories: 288

Fat: 1g

Carbohydrates: 60g

Fibre: 17g

Protein: 14g

Snack Recipes

here are ten snack recipes that are low in purines:

Roasted Chickpeas

Ingredients:

1 can chickpeas, drained and rinsed

1 tablespoon olive oil

1/2 teaspoon smoked paprika

1/2 teaspoon garlic powder

Salt and pepper, to taste

Instructions:

Preheat oven to 400°F (200°C) and line a baking sheet with parchment paper.

Pat chickpeas dry with a paper towel and remove any loose skins.

In a small bowl, mix olive oil, smoked paprika, garlic powder, salt, and pepper.

Toss chickpeas with the spice mixture until evenly coated.

Spread chickpeas in a single layer on the baking sheet and bake for 20-25 minutes, or until crispy and golden brown.

Remove from the oven and let cool for a few minutes before serving.

Nutrition Facts (per serving):

Calories: 130

Fat: 5g

Carbohydrates: 16g

Fibre: 4g

Protein: 5g

Greek Yogurt Dip with Veggies

Ingredients:

1 cup Greek yoghurt

1/2 teaspoon garlic powder

1/2 teaspoon dried dill

1/4 teaspoon onion powder

Salt and pepper, to taste

Carrot sticks, celery sticks, and/or cucumber slices, for serving

Instructions:

In a small bowl, mix Greek yoghurt, garlic powder, dried dill, onion powder, salt, and pepper.

Serve with carrot sticks, celery sticks, and/or cucumber slices for dipping.

Nutrition Facts (per serving):

Calories: 100

Fat: 1g

Carbohydrates: 8g

Fibre: 1g

Protein: 15g

Fruit Salad with Mint and Lime

Ingredients:

2 cups mixed fruit (such as strawberries, blueberries, pineapple, and/or mango), chopped

1 tablespoon honey

1 tablespoon lime juice

1 tablespoon chopped fresh mint leaves

Instructions:

In a medium bowl, mix chopped fruit, honey, lime juice, and fresh mint leaves.

Serve immediately or store in the refrigerator for up to 2 days.

Nutrition Facts (per serving):

Calories: 90

Fat: 0g

Carbohydrates: 23g

Fibre: 3g / Protein: 1g

Hummus and Veggie Sticks

Ingredients:

1 can of chickpeas, drained and rinsed

2 cloves of garlic, minced

3 tablespoons of tahini

2 tablespoons of lemon juice

1/4 teaspoon of cumin

Salt and pepper to taste

Carrots, celery, and cucumber sticks for dipping

Instructions:

In a food processor, combine the chickpeas, garlic, tahini, lemon juice, cumin, salt, and pepper.

Pulse until smooth and creamy, adding a tablespoon of water if necessary to reach desired consistency.

Serve with veggie sticks for dipping.

Nutrition Information:

Calories: 129

Carbohydrates: 14g

Protein: 6g

Fat: 6g

Saturated Fat: 1g

Sodium: 104mg

Fibre: 4g

Sugar: 2g

Baked Sweet Potato Chips

Ingredients:

2 sweet potatoes, thinly sliced

2 tablespoons of olive oil

Salt and pepper to taste

Instructions:

Preheat the oven to 375°F (190°C).

In a bowl, toss the sweet potato slices with olive oil, salt, and pepper.

Arrange the sweet potato slices in a single layer on a baking sheet lined with parchment paper.

Bake for 20-25 minutes or until crispy and golden brown.

Serve immediately.

Nutrition Information:

Calories: 139

Carbohydrates: 22g

Protein: 2g

Fat: 6g

Saturated Fat: 1g

Sodium: 99mg

Fibre: 3g

Sugar: 5g

Greek Yogurt Parfait

Ingredients:

1 cup of plain Greek yoghurt

1/2 cup of mixed berries

1/4 cup of granola

Instructions:

In a small bowl, layer the Greek yoghurt, mixed berries, and granola.

Repeat until all ingredients are used up.

Serve immediately.

Nutrition Information:

Calories: 234

Carbohydrates: 32g

Protein: 16g

Fat: 6g

Saturated Fat: 1g

Sodium: 57mg

Fibre: 5g

Sugar: 15g

Almond Butter and Banana Toast

Ingredients:

2 slices of whole-grain bread

2 tablespoons of almond butter

1 banana, sliced

Instructions:

Toast the bread slices until golden brown.

Spread each slice with 1 tablespoon of almond butter.

Top with sliced banana.

Serve immediately.

Nutrition Information:

Calories: 345

Carbohydrates: 49g

Protein: 11g

Fat: 14g

Saturated Fat: 1g

Sodium: 282mg

Fibre: 10g / Sugar: 16g

Carrot and Cucumber Sticks with Hummus

Ingredients:

2 medium-sized carrots, cut into sticks

1 medium-sized cucumber, cut into sticks

1/2 cup of hummus

Instructions:

Wash and cut the carrots and cucumber into sticks.

Place the hummus in a small bowl.

Serve the carrot and cucumber sticks with the hummus on the side for dipping.

Nutrition Facts:

Serving size: 1/2 cup of hummus with 1 cup of carrot and cucumber sticks

Calories: 135

Fat: 6g

Carbohydrates: 18g

Fibre: 6g

Protein: 5g

Greek Yogurt and Berries

Ingredients:

1 cup of plain Greek yoghurt

1/2 cup of mixed berries (such as strawberries, blueberries, and raspberries)

1 tbsp of honey (optional)

Instructions:

Rinse the berries and pat dry with a paper towel.

In a small bowl, mix the Greek yoghurt and honey (if using) until well combined.

Top the yoghurt with mixed berries.

Nutrition Facts:

Serving size: 1 cup of Greek yoghurt with 1/2 cup of mixed berries

Calories: 150 / Fat: 0g / Carbohydrates: 22g

Fibre: 3g / Protein: 16g

Dessert Recipes

Here are ten dessert recipes that are low in purines:

Mixed Berry Sorbet

Ingredients:

2 cups mixed berries (such as strawberries, blueberries, and raspberries)

1/2 cup water

1/2 cup sugar

1 tbsp fresh lemon juice

Instructions:

In a medium saucepan, combine water and sugar. Bring to a boil over medium heat, stirring until the sugar dissolves.

Add the mixed berries to the saucepan and cook for 5-7 minutes, stirring occasionally.

Remove from heat and let cool for 10 minutes.

Puree the mixture in a blender until smooth.

Stir in the fresh lemon juice.

Pour the mixture into a container and freeze for 4-6 hours, stirring occasionally, until firm.

Serve and enjoy!

Nutrition facts per serving (serves 4):

Calories: 96

Total fat: 0.2g

Saturated fat: 0g

Cholesterol: 0mg

Sodium: 0mg

Total Carbohydrates: 25g

Dietary Fiber: 3g

Sugars: 21g

Protein: 1g

Banana Oatmeal Cookies

Ingredients:

2 ripe bananas, mashed

1 cup rolled oats

1/4 cup chopped walnuts

1/4 cup dried cranberries

1/4 tsp cinnamon

1/4 tsp vanilla extract

Instructions:

Preheat the oven to 350°F (180°C). Line a baking
sheet with parchment paper.

In a mixing bowl, combine mashed bananas, rolled oats, chopped walnuts, dried cranberries, cinnamon, and vanilla extract. Stir until well combined.

Drop spoonfuls of the mixture onto the prepared baking sheet, spacing them 1 inch apart.

Bake for 15-20 minutes or until the cookies are golden brown.

Remove from the oven and let cool for 5 minutes.

Transfer the cookies to a wire rack and let them cool completely.

Serve and enjoy!

Nutrition facts per serving (serves 12):

Calories: 69

Total fat: 2.2g

Saturated fat: 0.3g

Cholesterol: 0mg

Sodium: 1mg

Total Carbohydrates: 12.3g

Dietary Fiber: 1.7g

Sugars: 5.5g

Protein: 1.6g

Grilled Peaches with Yogurt and Honey

Ingredients:

4 ripe peaches, halved and pitted

1 tbsp olive oil

1/2 cup plain Greek yoghurt

2 tbsp honey

1/4 cup chopped pecans

Instructions:

Preheat the grill to medium-high heat.

Brush the peach halves with olive oil.

Place the peaches on the grill, cut the side down, and cook for 3-4 minutes or until grill marks appear.

Flip the peaches and cook for an additional 2-3 minutes.

Remove the peaches from the grill and let cool for 5 minutes.

In a small bowl, whisk together the Greek yoghurt and honey.

Serve the grilled peaches with a dollop of the yoghurt mixture and a sprinkle of chopped pecans.

Enjoy!

Nutrition facts per serving (serves 4):

Calories: 163

Baked Pears with Honey and Walnuts

Ingredients:

4 ripe pears

2 tablespoons honey

1/4 cup chopped walnuts

1 teaspoon cinnamon

1/4 teaspoon nutmeg

1 tablespoon butter

Instructions:

Preheat oven to 375°F.

Cut pears in half and scoop out the core with a spoon.

Place the pears in a baking dish and drizzle with honey.

In a small bowl, mix walnuts, cinnamon, and nutmeg. Sprinkle the walnut mixture over the pears.

Cut the butter into small pieces and place them on top of the pears.

Bake for 30-40 minutes or until the pears are tender.

Serve warm.

Nutrition Information (per serving):

Calories: 165

Fat: 6g

Carbohydrates: 32g

Fibre: 6g

Protein: 2g

Strawberry Banana Smoothie

Ingredients:

1 cup fresh or frozen strawberries

1 ripe banana

1 cup almond milk

1 tablespoon honey

1/2 teaspoon vanilla extract

1/2 cup ice

Instructions:

Add all ingredients to a blender.

Blend until smooth.

Pour into a glass and enjoy!

Nutrition Information (per serving):

Calories: 170

Fat: 3g

Carbohydrates: 36g

Fibre: 5g

Protein: 3g

Chocolate Avocado Pudding

Ingredients:

2 ripe avocados

1/4 cup unsweetened cocoa powder

1/4 cup honey

1/4 cup almond milk

1/2 teaspoon vanilla extract

Instructions:

Cut avocados in half and remove the pit.

Scoop out the flesh and place it in a blender.

Add cocoa powder, honey, almond milk, and vanilla extract to the blender.

Blend until smooth and creamy.

Serve immediately or chill in the refrigerator for 30 minutes before serving.

Nutrition Information (per serving):

Calories: 220 / Fat: 13g / Fibre: 8g

Carbohydrates: 30g / Protein: 3g

Banana Oat Cookies

Ingredients:

2 ripe bananas, mashed

1 cup rolled oats

1/4 cup unsweetened shredded coconut

1/4 cup chopped walnuts

1/4 cup raisins

1 tsp cinnamon

1/2 tsp vanilla extract

Pinch of salt

Instructions:

Preheat oven to 350°F (180°C) and line a baking sheet with parchment paper.

In a bowl, mix mashed bananas, oats, coconut, walnuts, raisins, cinnamon, vanilla extract, and salt.

Using a spoon or cookie scoop, drop the mixture onto the prepared baking sheet, and gently press down to flatten slightly.

Bake for 15-20 minutes, until lightly golden brown.

Let cool for a few minutes before transferring to a wire rack to cool completely.

Nutrition facts (per serving):

Calories: 120

Fat: 5g

Carbohydrates: 18g

Fibre: 3g

Sugar: 7g

Protein: 3g

Chia Pudding with Fresh Berries

Ingredients:

1 cup unsweetened almond milk

1/4 cup chia seeds

1 tbsp honey or maple syrup

1/2 tsp vanilla extract

1 cup mixed fresh berries (e.g. strawberries, blueberries, raspberries)

Instructions:

In a bowl, whisk together almond milk, chia seeds, honey or maple syrup, and vanilla extract until well combined.

Cover and refrigerate for at least 2 hours, or overnight, until thickened.

When ready to serve, divide the chia pudding into 4 bowls, and top with fresh berries.

Nutrition facts (per serving):

Calories: 110

Fat: 5g

Carbohydrates: 15g

Fibre: 9g

Sugar: 6g

Protein: 4g

Baked Pears with Honey and Walnuts

Ingredients:

2 ripe pears, halved and cored

2 tablespoons honey

1/4 cup chopped walnuts

1/2 teaspoon cinnamon

1/4 teaspoon nutmeg

Instructions:

Preheat oven to 375°F (190°C).

Place pear halves on a baking sheet, and cut side up.

Drizzle honey over each pear half.

Sprinkle chopped walnuts, cinnamon, and nutmeg over the pears.

Bake for 20-25 minutes, or until pears are soft and walnuts are toasted.

Serve warm.

Nutrition facts (per serving):

Calories: 165

Fat: 7g

Carbohydrates: 27g

Protein: 2g

Sodium: 2mg

Fibre: 4g

Sugar: 20g

Chia Seed Pudding

Ingredients:

1/4 cup chia seeds

1 cup almond milk

1 tablespoon honey

1/4 teaspoon vanilla extract

1/4 teaspoon cinnamon

Fresh fruit for topping (optional)

Instructions:

In a medium-sized bowl, mix chia seeds, almond milk, honey, vanilla extract, and cinnamon.

Stir until all ingredients are well combined.

Cover and refrigerate for at least 2 hours, or overnight.

When ready to serve, give the pudding a good stir and top with fresh fruit, if desired.

Nutrition facts (per serving):

Calories: 160

Fat: 8g

Carbohydrates: 18g

Protein: 5g

Sodium: 90mg

Fibre: 10g

Sugar: 7g

Berry Yogurt Parfait

Ingredients:

1 cup plain Greek yoghurt

1/2 cup mixed berries (fresh or frozen)

2 tablespoons chopped almonds

1 tablespoon honey

1/4 teaspoon vanilla extract

Instructions:

In a small bowl, mix Greek yoghurt, honey, and vanilla extract.

In a separate bowl, toss together mixed berries and chopped almonds.

To assemble the parfait, layer half of the yoghurt mixture, followed by half of the berry mixture in a glass or jar.

Repeat with another layer of yoghurt and berries.

Serve immediately.

Nutrition facts (per serving):

Calories: 220

Fat: 9g

Carbohydrates: 21g

Protein: 18g

Sodium: 65mg

Fibre: 4g

Sugar: 13g.

CHAPTER FIVE

MEAL PLANNING AND PREPARATION TIPS

Tips for Meal planning with the Low Purine Diet

Meal planning might be difficult with the low purine diet, but with a little foresight, it can be a breeze. Here are some pointers for good low-purine diet meal planning:

Make a plan: Take the time to plan your meals ahead of time. This will help you keep on track and ensure that you have healthy, low-purine alternatives on hand at all times.

Maintain Simplicity: Avoid overcomplicating things by attempting to prepare complex meals. Adhere to basic, healthful, and quick-to-prepare choices.

Concentrate on fresh, healthy Foods: Include fresh fruits and vegetables, lean meats, and whole grains in your meals. These meals are high in minerals and critical vitamins while being low in purines.

Experiment with Herbs and Spices: To add taste without introducing purines, use a variety of herbs and spices while cooking low-purine meals. To enhance taste, try basil, oregano, rosemary, and thyme.

Meal Planning: Plan your meals for the week ahead of time. This will save you time and guarantee that you always have healthy alternatives on hand when you need them.

Drink lots of water throughout the day to help flush out uric acid and avoid gout flare-ups.

Moderation is essential: Although it is important to adhere to low-purine alternatives, it is equally critical to exercise moderation. Instead of depriving yourself of the foods you like, limit your quantities and eat in moderation.

You may effectively plan and prepare nutritious, low-purine meals that will keep you feeling fantastic and lower your risk of gout flare-ups by following these guidelines.

Planning low-purine meals in advance

Planning low-purine meals ahead of time will help you keep to your low-purine diet while also saving time on hectic weekdays. Here are some pointers for planning ahead of time low purine meals:

Plan your Meals: Before you begin cooking, make a plan for the week's meals. This will ensure that you have all of the necessary components and will save you time over the week.

Cook in bulk: Preparing in bulk low-purine dishes might save you time and provide you with leftovers for the week. Soups, stews, and casseroles are excellent choices for big amounts.

Make use of Meal Prep Containers: Purchase meal prep containers that are portioned out for each meal. This will help you stick to your portion proportions and make it easier to grab a meal on the run.

Freeze individual parts of low-purine meals: If you're creating a big quantity of a low-purine dish, freeze individual portions for later use. This will save you time throughout the week and guarantee that you have a nutritious dinner on hand at all times.

Preparing components like veggies, cereals, and meats ahead of time will help you save time throughout the week. Prepare veggies, grains, and meats ahead of time so that you can quickly put together a meal throughout the week.

You may keep on track with your diet and save time during the hectic weekdays by taking the effort to prepare low-purine meals ahead of time.

How to include low-purine foods in your regular diet

Adding low-purine meals into your daily routine will help you manage gout and live a healthy lifestyle.

Here are some ideas to help you include low-purine foods into your everyday diet:

Begin by compiling a list of low-purine foods: When you begin adding low-purine meals into your daily routine, you need first to understand which foods are low in purines. Create a list of low-purine foods and have it ready for when you're grocery shopping or meal planning.

Plan your meals: Preparing your meals in advance may help you guarantee that you're eating a range of low-purine foods. Plan your meals for the week using your list of low-purine foods, making sure to include a variety of fruits, vegetables, nutritious grains, and lean meats.

Batch cook Low Purine Foods: Making low-purine meals ahead of time may save you time and make sticking to a low-purine diet simpler. Make big quantities of reduced purine soups, stews, and casseroles and freeze individual portions for later warming.

Explore new recipes: Experimenting with new low-purine dishes will help you find new foods and tastes you like. Search for low-purine recipes online or in cookbooks, and try various herbs, spices, and seasonings to provide taste without introducing purines.

Have a supply of nutritious Snacks: Snacking on low-purine foods will help you feel full and content between meals. Have nutritious snacks on hand, such as fresh fruits and vegetables and almonds, for when you need a fast snack.

By implementing these strategies into your daily routine, you may make it simpler to adhere to a reduced purine diet and successfully manage your gout symptoms.

4 Week Sample Meal Plan

Here is a 4-week sample meal plan for the low-purine diet:

Week 1:

Monday:

Breakfast: Spinach and Feta Omelette with Whole Grain Toast

Snack: Carrot Sticks with Hummus

Lunch: Tuna Salad with Avocado and Whole Grain Crackers

Snack: Apple Slices with Almond Butter

Dinner: Grilled Chicken Breast with Quinoa Pilaf and Roasted Vegetables

Tuesday:

Breakfast: Greek Yogurt with Mixed Berries and Chia Seeds

Snack: Hard Boiled Egg

Lunch: Lentil Soup with Whole Grain Roll

Snack: Orange Slices

Dinner: Baked Salmon with Brown Rice and Steamed Broccoli

Wednesday:

Breakfast: Banana Pancakes with Maple Syrup and Turkey Bacon

Snack: Trail Mix (Mixed Nuts, Dried Fruit, and Seeds)

Lunch: Turkey and Swiss Cheese Sandwich with Whole Grain Bread and Side Salad

Snack: Edamame

Dinner: Beef Stir-Fry with Brown Rice and Mixed Vegetables

Thursday:

Breakfast: Oatmeal with Walnuts and Cinnamon

Snack: Cottage Cheese with Pineapple Chunks

Lunch: Grilled Chicken Caesar Salad

Snack: Grapes

Dinner: Stuffed Bell Peppers with Ground Turkey and Quinoa

Friday:

Breakfast: Egg and Cheese Bagel Sandwich

Snack: Greek Yogurt with Granola

Lunch: Tuna and White Bean Salad with Whole Grain Crackers

Snack: Mango Slices

Dinner: Lemon Garlic Shrimp with Zucchini Noodles

Saturday:

Breakfast: Whole Wheat Waffles with Peanut Butter and Fresh Berries

Snack: Celery Sticks with Peanut Butter

Lunch: Grilled Vegetable Wrap with a Side Salad

Snack: Blueberry Smoothie

Dinner: Beef Chili with Whole Grain Bread and Side Salad

Sunday:

Breakfast: Breakfast Burrito with Scrambled Eggs, Salsa, and Avocado

Snack: Hard Boiled Egg

Lunch: Chickpea Salad with Whole Grain Pita Bread

Snack: Kiwi Slices

Dinner: Grilled Chicken Kebabs with Couscous and Grilled Vegetables

Week 2:

Monday

Breakfast: Greek yoghurt with sliced strawberries and chopped walnuts

Lunch: Tuna salad with mixed greens, cherry tomatoes, and cucumber

Snack: Apple slices with almond butter

Dinner: Grilled chicken breast with roasted asparagus and quinoa

Tuesday

Breakfast: Spinach and mushroom omelette with whole wheat toast

Lunch: Lentil soup with a side salad

Snack: Carrot sticks with hummus

Dinner: Baked salmon with roasted Brussels sprouts and brown rice

Wednesday

Breakfast: Overnight oats with blueberries and chia seeds

Lunch: Quinoa salad with roasted vegetables and feta cheese

Snack: Edamame

Dinner: Grilled portobello mushroom burger with sweet potato fries

Thursday

Breakfast: Scrambled eggs with sautéed spinach and whole wheat toast

Lunch: Grilled chicken Caesar salad

Snack: Trail mix

Dinner: Baked chicken thigh with steamed broccoli and quinoa

Friday

Breakfast: Avocado toast with smoked salmon

Lunch: Greek salad with grilled chicken

Snack: Roasted chickpeas

Dinner: Vegetable stir-fry with brown rice

Saturday

Breakfast: Banana pancakes with almond butter

Lunch: Grilled shrimp skewers with mixed greens and cherry tomatoes

Snack: Fresh fruit salad

Dinner: Baked cod with roasted root vegetables and quinoa

Sunday

Breakfast: Veggie omelette with whole wheat toast

Lunch: Lentil and vegetable soup with a side salad

Snack: Raw vegetables with tzatziki dip

Dinner: Grilled chicken breast with roasted sweet potatoes and green beans

Week 3:

Monday

Breakfast: Greek yoghurt with sliced peaches and chopped almonds

Lunch: Turkey and cheese sandwich with raw veggies

Snack: Fresh fruit

Dinner: Vegetable stir-fry with tofu and brown rice

Tuesday

Breakfast: Oatmeal with mixed berries and chopped walnuts

Lunch: Greek salad with grilled shrimp

Snack: Roasted almonds

Dinner: Baked salmon with roasted broccoli and quinoa

Wednesday

Breakfast: Veggie scramble with whole wheat toast

Lunch: Grilled chicken Caesar salad

Snack: Raw veggies with hummus

Dinner: Lentil shepherd's pie

Thursday

Breakfast: Smoothie bowl with mixed berries and chia seeds

Lunch: Tuna salad with mixed greens, cherry tomatoes, and cucumber

Snack: Hard-boiled egg

Dinner: Grilled portobello mushroom burger with sweet potato fries

Friday

Breakfast: Avocado toast with hard-boiled egg

Lunch: Quinoa salad with roasted vegetables and feta cheese

Snack: Fresh fruit

Dinner: Baked chicken thigh with steamed asparagus and brown rice

Saturday

Breakfast: Banana pancakes with almond butter

Lunch: Lentil and vegetable soup with a side salad

Snack: Roasted chickpeas

Dinner: Baked cod with roasted root vegetables and quinoa

Sunday

Breakfast: Veggie omelette with whole wheat toast

Lunch: Grilled shrimp skewers with mixed greens and cherry tomatoes

Snack: Fresh fruit salad

Dinner: Grilled chicken breast with roasted sweet potatoes and green beans

Week 4

Monday

Breakfast: Scrambled eggs with spinach, whole wheat toast, and a banana

Snack: Greek yoghurt with fresh blueberries

Lunch: Grilled chicken breast with roasted vegetables (zucchini, bell peppers, onions) and quinoa

Snack: Apple slices with almond butter

Dinner: Broiled salmon with steamed asparagus and wild rice

Tuesday

Breakfast: Smoothie made with Greek yoghurt, frozen mixed berries, spinach, and almond milk

Snack: Carrots and celery sticks with hummus

Lunch: Turkey and avocado wrap with lettuce and tomato on a whole wheat tortilla, served with a side salad

Snack: Orange slices

Dinner: Baked chicken thighs with roasted Brussels sprouts and sweet potatoes

Wednesday

Breakfast: Oatmeal with sliced banana, chopped walnuts, and a drizzle of honey

Snack: Homemade trail mix (almonds, cashews, raisins, and dried apricots)

Lunch: Lentil and vegetable soup with a side of whole-wheat bread

Snack: Pear slices with cheese

Dinner: Grilled flank steak with roasted root vegetables (carrots, parsnips, and beets) and a side salad

Thursday

Breakfast: Breakfast burrito with scrambled eggs, black beans, avocado, and salsa on a whole wheat tortilla

Snack: Cottage cheese with fresh pineapple

Lunch: Tuna salad (made with Greek yoghurt instead of mayo) on a bed of mixed greens with cherry tomatoes and cucumber

Snack: Kiwi slices

Dinner: Vegetarian chilli with a side of brown rice and a mixed greens salad

Friday

Breakfast: Veggie omelette (with onions, mushrooms, and bell peppers) and a slice of whole wheat toast

Snack: Homemade energy balls (made with rolled oats, peanut butter, and honey)

Lunch: Grilled shrimp with quinoa and a side of steamed green beans

Snack: Homemade guacamole with cucumber slices

Dinner: Grilled salmon with roasted Brussels sprouts and a side salad

Saturday

Breakfast: Whole grain pancakes with fresh berries and a drizzle of maple syrup

Snack: Plain popcorn

Lunch: Chicken Caesar salad (made with Greek yoghurt instead of dressing) and a whole wheat pita

Snack: Mango slices with Greek yoghurt

Dinner: Beef stir-fry (with broccoli, carrots, and onions) and brown rice

Sunday

Breakfast: Greek yoghurt parfait with granola and mixed berries

Snack: Roasted chickpeas

Lunch: Grilled chicken breast with sweet potato wedges and a side salad

Snack: Hard-boiled egg with cherry tomatoes

Dinner: Baked cod with steamed green beans and a side of wild rice

CHAPTER SIX

LIFESTYLE MODIFICATIONS FOR GOUT MANAGEMENT

The importance of exercise in gout management

Exercise may help decrease inflammation, enhance joint mobility, and encourage weight reduction, all of which can assist with gout management. Frequent exercise may also enhance general health and well-being, lowering the chance of acquiring other chronic disorders that might aggravate gout symptoms, such as heart disease and diabetes.

Numerous sorts of exercise may be useful to persons suffering from gout, including:

Aerobic Exercise: Aerobic activity, such as brisk walking, jogging, cycling, or swimming, may improve cardiovascular health and encourage weight reduction, all of which can help lessen gout symptoms.

Strength Training: Strength training may assist enhance muscular strength and joint stability, lowering the risk of joint damage and improving joint function.

Flexibility Exercises: Stretching and other flexibility exercises may assist increase joint mobility and decreasing stiffness, which can be especially useful for people with gout who have joint discomfort and restricted movement.

Before beginning an exercise program, it is important to contact a healthcare expert, especially if you have underlying health concerns that may be impacted by exercise. To prevent increasing gout symptoms, begin cautiously and gradually increase the intensity and duration of activity. Also, keeping hydrated and wearing suitable footwear might help reduce gout episodes when exercising.

Tips for reducing stress and improving sleep Since stress and a lack of sleep may aggravate gout symptoms, it is important to make steps to minimize stress and enhance sleep quality. Here are some pointers:

Practice Relaxation Techniques: Participate in relaxation practices such as deep breathing, meditation, yoga, or tai chi to assist decrease stress.

Exercise Regularly: Frequent exercise may assist to decrease stress and enhance sleep quality. Spend at least 30 minutes every day, most days of the week, walking, running, swimming, cycling, or weight training.

Create a consistent sleep schedule: Try to go to bed and get up at the same time every day, especially on weekends. Creating a consistent sleep regimen might assist in training your body to sleep more peacefully.

Avoid stimulants: Avoid ingesting stimulants such as coffee and nicotine close to bedtime since they might disrupt sleep quality.

Make your sleeping environment peaceful: Make sure your sleeping environment is relaxing. Maintain a dark, quiet, and cool environment in the room, and invest in a comfortable mattress and pillows.

Minimize screen time: Avoid using screens such as TV, laptops, and cell phones for at least an hour before going to bed. Screen blue light may disrupt sleep by decreasing the generation of melatonin, a hormone that governs sleep.

Consult a healthcare expert: If your stress and sleep issues continue, consult a healthcare professional about various solutions such as counselling, medication, or therapy.

By implementing these suggestions into your daily routine, you may help control stress and increase sleep quality, both of which can assist with gout symptoms.

How to Keep a Healthy Weight on a Low Purine Diet

Keeping a healthy weight is critical for gout management since being overweight or obese increases the likelihood of gout episodes. These are some ideas for maintaining a healthy weight while on the reduced purine diet:

Eat a balanced Diet: Have a balanced diet that contains a range of low-purine foods such as vegetables, fruits, whole grains, and lean protein sources. Avoid processed and high-calorie foods that might contribute to weight gain.

Portion control: Portion control is essential for weight loss. Utilize smaller plates, prevent second helpings, and weigh your meals to verify you're eating the correct portion proportions.

Reduce your alcohol consumption: Alcohol contains a lot of calories and might lead to weight gain. Also, alcohol intake is a typical cause of gout episodes. If you must drink, do it in moderation and pick low-calorie beverages such as light beer or wine.

Drink enough Water: Consuming plenty of water might make you feel full and lower your appetite. Drink at least eight glasses of water every day and avoid sugary beverages like soda and juice.

Exercise regularly: Exercise is important for weight loss and may also help decrease stress and improve sleep quality. Include at least 30 minutes of moderate-intensity activity in your daily regimens, such as brisk walking or cycling.

Contact a trained dietitian: A registered dietitian can assist you in developing a tailored meal plan that fulfils your nutritional requirements as well as your weight control objectives while also managing your gout symptoms.

To summarize, keeping a healthy weight is critical to controlling gout and minimizing the risk of gout episodes. A low-purine diet may help you manage your gout, and combining regular physical exercise and stress-reduction tactics can help you lose weight and improve your overall health.

To be healthy on the low-purine diet, it's crucial to choose nutrient-dense, low-calorie meals and watch your portion sizes. Healthy protein sources, such as lentils, tofu, and lean meats, as well as lots of fruits and vegetables, may help increase satiety and offer necessary nutrients.

Limiting high-calorie, high-fat, and processed meals, which may lead to weight gain and increase the risk of gout attacks, is also vital. Keeping hydrated and avoiding sugary beverages may also aid in weight management and general health.

Overall, keeping a healthy weight and adhering to a low-purine diet may be an effective method to control gout and enhance overall health. You may help your body and lower your chance of gout attacks by implementing good eating habits, frequent physical exercise, and stress reduction strategies into your daily routine. Contact a trained dietitian or healthcare practitioner to build a specific strategy for gout management and weight maintenance.

CHAPTER SEVEN:

SUMMARY AND NEXT STEPS

Recap of the low purine diet and how it helps manage gout

In essence, the low purine diet is an eating plan that reduces the number of purines in the diet, which may help control gout. Purines are included in a variety of foods and may raise uric acid levels in the body, causing gout symptoms. Gout patients may lower their risk of flare-ups and control their symptoms by reducing high-purine meals and opting for low-purine ones.

A low-purine diet should contain lots of fruits and vegetables, and lean proteins, and avoid or restrict high-purine items such as organ meats, shellfish, and some kinds of fish. Meal planning and preparation may also aid in adhering to a reduced purine diet and avoiding the temptation to consume high-purine items.

Keeping a healthy weight is also crucial for gout management since excess weight may exacerbate gout symptoms. Weight management and general health may be improved by combining a reduced purine diet with regular exercise and stress reduction measures.

Before beginning a new diet or making substantial changes to your eating habits, contact a healthcare provider or certified dietitian, particularly if you have a medical condition such as gout. They may provide tailored advice and assistance to help you manage your symptoms and improve your overall health.

The Significance of Self-care and Symptom Monitoring
Self-care and symptom monitoring are critical components of gout management. This involves maintaining your general health by eating a well-balanced diet, exercising regularly, managing stress, getting adequate sleep, and keeping a healthy weight. It is also critical to keep track of your symptoms, such as joint discomfort and

inflammation, and to seek medical assistance as needed.

Keeping note of your symptoms might assist you in identifying triggers and making required lifestyle or pharmaceutical modifications. It is also critical to collaborate closely with your healthcare practitioner to build an effective treatment plan and to follow up frequently.

Moreover, exercising self-care may enhance your overall quality of life and assist you in managing the emotional toll that comes with living with a chronic disease. This may involve participating in things that offer you pleasure, receiving assistance from loved ones, and developing healthy coping mechanisms for stress and anxiety.

Ultimately, self-care and symptom monitoring are critical in treating gout and enhancing overall health and well-being.

Resources and tools for ongoing support and information

For continued support and information about the low purine diet and gout therapy, there are various sites and tools available. Such examples are:

Dietitians and Nutritionists: These healthcare experts may provide individualized guidance and help when it comes to designing a low-purine meal plan and implementing dietary modifications.

Gout Support Groups: Participating in a support group may create a feeling of community while also allowing people to learn from others who are also dealing with gout.

Internet Resources: The Arthritis Foundation and the Gout and Uric Acid Education Society are two organizations that give information and support to those who have gout.

Mobile Applications: A variety of apps are available to assist people to track their symptoms, monitor their food and activities, and manage their medication. Gout Central, Gout Diary, and My Gout are other popular choices.

Books: "The Gout Solution" by Richard L. Becker and "Beating Gout" by Victor Konshin are two publications that give knowledge and assistance on controlling gout.

Individuals may remain educated and empowered in their gout treatment journey by using this information and tools.

Appendix: Resources and Commonly Asked Questions

Commonly Asked Questions:

What are some Purine-rich Foods to avoid?

Organ meats (liver, kidney, etc.), game meats (venison, rabbit, etc.), seafood (anchovies, sardines, mussels, etc.), and certain vegetables are high in purine (spinach, asparagus, mushrooms, etc.).

Can I have meat while on a Low Purine Diet?

Yes, you can consume meat on a low-purine diet, but pick lean meats and restrict your intake of high-purine foods like organ meats and game meats.

Can I have wine while on a Low Purine Diet?

On a reduced purine diet, alcohol should be restricted or avoided since it may increase the risk of gout episodes. Purines are notably abundant in beer and strong liquor.

Is there anything that may assist with Gout?

Certain supplements, such as vitamin C, may be beneficial in reducing gout symptoms. Nevertheless, it is important to consult with your doctor before beginning any supplements to verify that they are both safe and helpful for you.

Resources:

The Gout and Uric Acid Education Association is an organization committed to improving gout awareness and giving services to those suffering from the ailment.

The Arthritis Foundation is a non-profit organization that educates and supports individuals suffering from arthritis, especially gout.

The National Institute of Arthritis and Musculoskeletal and Skin Disorders is a federal institution that conducts research and offers information to those suffering from arthritis and other musculoskeletal disorders.

The American College of Rheumatology is a rheumatology professional organization that gives information and support to persons suffering from arthritis, particularly gout.

MyFitnessPal is a free app that may help you track your food and control your calorie consumption to maintain a healthy weight, which is essential for gout management.